The Making of a
Joyful Mother Workbook

The Making of a Joyful Mother Workbook

A SPIRITUAL JOURNEY FOR WOMEN EXPERIENCING INFERTILITY

Kimberly Webb

iUniverse, Inc.
New York Lincoln Shanghai

The Making of a Joyful Mother Workbook
A Spiritual Journey for Women Experiencing Infertility

iUniverse books may be ordered through booksellers or by contacting:

iUniverse
2021 Pine Lake Road, Suite 100
Lincoln, NE 68512
www.iuniverse.com
1-800-Authors (1-800-288-4677)

The views expressed in this work are solely those of the author and do not necessarily reflect the views of the publisher, and the publisher hereby disclaims any responsibility for them.

ISBN: 978-0-595-43698-9 (pbk)
ISBN: 978-0-595-88032-4 (ebk)

Printed in the United States of America

Psalms 113:9

"He makes the barren women abide in the house,
as a joyful mother of children. Praise the Lord."

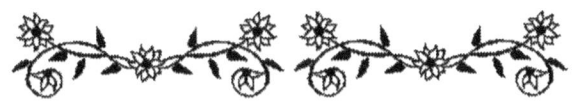

Contents

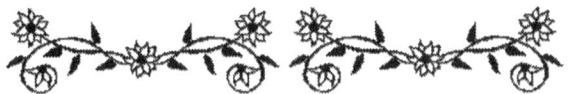

Acknowledgements

Thank you God for giving me a purpose and having patience with me. Thank you Jesus Christ for continuing to love me in spite of me. Thank you for blessing me with the gift of Kendal.

I want to give special thanks to my husband, Steven for his tireless efforts in editing and proofing this workbook. Thank you for loving me through good times and bad. Thank you for continuing to be my best friend and believing in God's vision for me. I thank God for giving you to me. You are my champion, my advocate. You see things in me that I don't always see. Thank you for causing me to look deeper.

Thanks to my parents for watching Kendal countless Sundays which helped me complete this workbook. Thanks so much for being the best grandparents in the world. We love you!

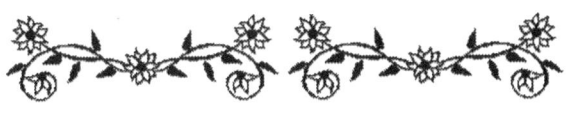

I

The Daughter's Struggle with Infertility

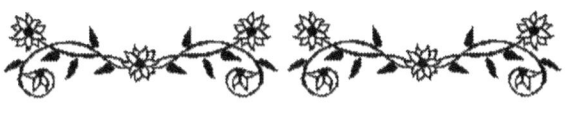

1

Day of Dependence

Proverbs 3:5 "Trust in the Lord with all your heart and do not lean on your own understanding. In all your ways acknowledge Him and He will direct your paths."

In our society, we are taught to be independent. We make our own decisions and march to our own beat. It's not so in the kingdom of God; God wants us to be dependent upon Him instead of dependent upon ourselves. This is a contradiction to the way the world sees life, and for many, it's a difficult transition. However, with time and prayer, the transition can occur. This workbook was written from a journey perspective and each chapter in Part I is a different road, fork, u-turn, or highway that guides you closer to the desired end of the journey—a street called "Destiny." But before we arrive at the last stop on the journey, we will travel on the main road for most of our trip. The main road is called the "Road to Fruitfulness." As we begin our journey, we will make a right turn on the street, "Day of Dependence," before proceeding onward. →

Analyze your life and write (3) three areas of your life (job, marriage or etc.) where you believe that you developed the perfect plan.

Examples: At the age of 23, I plan to apply for the management training program at my job.
Five years ago, my plan was to move out of this starter home and buy a new home with more space.

1) _____
_____.
2) _____
_____.
3) _____
_____.

From these (3) three areas, pick one area that did not go according as planned and explain your thoughts and feelings regarding the unfulfilled plan.

_____
_____
_____.

Did you try and help God complete your perfect plan?   Yes or No
If yes, explain in one sentence, how you tried to help God?

_____
_____.

Did your effort help or hurt the situation?

_____
_____
_____.

Jeremiah 29:11, For I know the plans I have for you, declares the Lord, plans for welfare and not for calamity to give you a future and a hope.

Oftentimes, we spend hours, sometimes days, developing plans for our lives and we feel our plans are perfect for us. As we begin to implement them, we are sometimes surprised at the outcome because they don't always turn out the way we planned. There is nothing wrong with planning as long as you realize that your plan is just that—your plan. As the scripture above states, God has plans for us and our plans must be in alignment with His plan. Submitting our plans to Him demonstrates our dependence on Him and helps us to realize

His sovereignty, especially when He decides to alter or change our plans according to His perfect will for our lives.

Explain in one sentence, how you tried to help God solve the issue of infertility in your life?

_____

_____.

In your own words, define independence and dependence

_____

_____

_____.

During my journey with infertility, God taught me some very important lessons on leading a life dependent on Him and leading an independent life separate and apart from Him. Sad to say, the beginning of my journey was spent as an independent Christian, acknowledging the Father, but not completely being dependent on Him. After a short time, God demonstrated to me, my first lesson—that I have many limitations when I am functioning independent of God.

Listed are areas I examined during my independence stage with God. Review these choices and check all of the areas where you perform independent of God.

Job Responsibilities	Household tasks	Friendships	Vacation
Health	Purchases/Finances	Entertainment	Family Size

Why do you think you are not consulting God in these areas? Check all that apply.

These areas belong to me	God is not interested
These areas are too minor to involve God	I can handle these areas myself

One of the first things we must realize in our quest for dependence on God is that all areas of our life **belong** to Him. God is **concerned** about and **interested** in all aspects of our life. The Bible says that *I can do nothing apart from God (John 15:5)*. I have found that submitting something as simple as my agenda for the day to Lord, inclusive of tasks, relationships and decisions allows everything to flow much smoother than if I tried to tackle all of it myself. It seems that I am less frustrated and frazzled because God is managing and prioritizing everything about me and my day.

Recognize the areas of your life that are independent of God and begin to submit them to Him now. Make a list of them and choose to bring them into His perfect sovereignty. After completing your list, pray to God ask Him to forgive you for being independent and show you how to be dependent on Him for these and all areas of your life.

1._____
2._____
3._____
4._____

The second lesson I learned about being independent of God is that God wants us to cry out to Him. I know many of you are saying, "I have already been crying out to God," and I don't doubt that you have. But, was it a cry for dependence on Him or just a cry for Him to answer your prayer for a baby? There is a big difference. We have all shed tears to God because our hearts are heavy and our arms are empty, but how many have cried out to God to show us how to depend on Him for our gift?

Let's do an inventory. Write all of the ways you've asked God to teach you how to be dependent on Him.

1. _____
2. _____
3. _____

Let's take it a step further, name all the people you talked to (cried out to), when you first found out that you had some infertility challenges.

1. _____   4. _____
2. _____   5. _____
3. _____   6. _____

† Did God make your list? Was He first, last or not on the list at all? It makes you think: if I can do nothing apart from Him, then why am I consulting other people regarding my infertility? This workbook is designed to answer some of these questions and cause you to pursue and recognize God's position in your life. Having a proper perspective of Him will aid you as you walk with Him through this journey of infertility.

> *Recognize your limitations Realize your position Rely on God for everything*

When we begin depending on God, He sends us glimmers of hope. A glimmer is a faint light that is sometimes quick and fleeting. A glimmer of hope is an encouraging word, prophecy or an act of faith that comes from a person(s) who believes for and with you for your child. Fortunately for us, with life's constant struggles, God frequently provides us with these glimmers. As I discussed in Chapter 1 of my book, "The Making of a Joyful Mother," God sent me three glimmers of hope, all were from prophetic words and packed with encouragement, strength and faith.

Describe your (3) three glimmers of hope and explain the reason God sent them to you.

1. _____
   _____
   _____
   _____.

2. _____

   _____

   _____.

   _____

3. _____

   _____

   _____

   _____.

It is important to write down these glimmers of hope and hold onto them, because they help to increase your faith and are reminders that God has not forgotten about you. You can use these glimmers as weapons of war, when Satan wants you to question your ability to have a child. If you have not received any glimmers of hope, pray and ask God to send them to you.

Sarah's Independence vs. Hannah's Dependence

In Chapter 1 of "The Making of a Joyful Mother," we discussed Sarah's independence of God and Hannah's dependence upon God. What do you think would have happened if Sarah had not taken her infertility into her own hands? (Refer to the story recorded in Genesis chapter 16 of Abraham, Sarah and Hagar.)

_____

_____

_____

_____.

What do you think Sarah learned by acting independent of God?

_____

_____

_____

_____.

What were the lifelong ramifications of Sarah's decision?

_____

_____

_____.

Read 1 Samuel Chapter 1. Then read Hannah's prayer to God found in 1 Samuel 1:11 and write it below.

_____

_____

_____

_____.

Check all of Hannah's attributes that are exhibited in her prayer.

Meekness	Self-reliant	Humble	Reverence for God
Impatient	Specific	Aggressive	Dependent

Why do you think God answered Hannah's prayer?

_____

_____

_____

_____.

Are you most like Sarah?
     Yes   No

If yes, list the attributes that you possess that are most like Sarah.

_____

_____.

Are you most like Hannah?
     Yes   No

If yes, list the attributes that you possess that are most like Hannah.

_____

_____

_____.

Or, are you a little of both?
     Yes   No

If yes, explain why?

_____

_____

_____.

Suggested Prayer:

Lord,

I come to you acknowledging that you are Lord over all of my life. I repent from asserting my independence separate and apart from You. I am sorry; please forgive me for my actions. I am dependent upon You for everything, even little things I take for granted. Reveal areas in my life where I have acted independent of You. I have been independent for so long, please show me how to be dependant on You. I love You and want to glorify You. I am totally dependent on You to bring about this blessing of a child from my womb. I am no longer relying on other's advice; it's just You and me. Please give me a child so that I can give him/her back to You to be used by You as You please.

Your Daughter,
In Jesus Name,
Amen

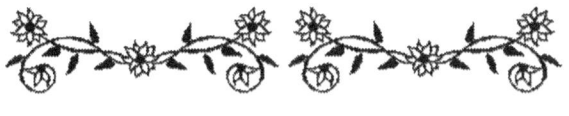

2

Desire vs. God's Design

Psalms 37:4 "Delight yourself in the Lord;
and He will give you the desires of your heart"

"Day of Dependence" had a lot of winding curves, and at times, it was difficult to navigate. But I am sure you were able to travel safely. As you are walking, you see ahead, "Desire vs. God's Design" directing you onto another street. As you continue there are signs ahead that say, "Turn right where you will find fruit and pecan trees straight ahead." You think to yourself, "I am going to stop and pick up some apples, pears, oranges and maybe even some pecans." Finally, you turn on the street, but you can barely see the trees; they are so far away and spread so far apart. From where you are walking, they seem way out of reach. Of course, if you had designed this tree patch, you would have planted the trees much closer to the roadway. But, you were not given the authority to architecturally align the trees as you please; instead, someone with more authority designed and planted the trees. As you walk on this long journey, you may be tempted to ask yourself, "Why do I want this fruit?" It sounds like a silly question, but why? Could it be that something way down deep desires the fruit? You are probably unable to explain it, but the fact is, you know that you want.

Write Psalms 103: 19

_____

_____

_____

_____.

Define in your own words sovereignty

_____

_____.

Why do you think God gives us desires?

_____

_____.

Why don't we have authority to carry out many of our desires?

_____

_____.

Why are we subject to God's design for our lives?

_____

_____.

What would life be like if we were allowed to design our own lives?

_____

_____.

Why is it important for God's authority to rule over us?

_____

_____.

Let's look at an example of two sisters in Genesis 29-30, both wish to carry out their own desires instead of following God's design for their lives.

This sibling rivalry between Leah and Rachel involves the love of a man, birth of a child, and love & praise for God.

Read this story and analyze each sister's desires and God's design for their lives. Answer the below questions.

1. Which sister is the eldest sister? _____

2. How do you think Leah felt about Jacob's desire for Rachel?

    _____
    _____
    _____.

3. Describe Leah's physical attributes and upbringing.

    _____
    _____
    _____.

4. Describe Rachel's physical attributes and upbringing.

    _____
    _____
    _____.

5. Why do you think Rachel was jealous of Leah?

    _____
    _____
    _____.

6. Why do you think Leah was jealous of Rachel?

    _____
    _____.

7. List the motives for Leah and Rachel wanting to get pregnant?
    Leah—_____
    Rachel—_____

8. What is your motive for wanting to get pregnant?

    _____

    _____.

9. Why do you think God opened Leah's womb?

    _____

    _____

    _____.

10. Was Leah's desire for Jacob's love greater than her love for God?

          Yes   No

11. After Leah had her fourth child, what was her response to God? Why?

    _____

    _____.

12. Why did Rachel blame Jacob for her inability to conceive?

    _____

    _____

    _____.

13. What was Jacob's response to Rachel?

    _____

    _____

    _____.

14. What do you think God was trying to teach Rachel?

    _____

    _____

    _____.

15. What do you think God was trying to teach Leah?

_____

_____

_____.

16. What has God taught you through Rachel and Leah?

_____

_____

_____

_____

_____.

17. Read Proverbs 3:5-6 and write it down.

_____

_____

_____

_____

_____

_____.

Check each statement that demonstrates trust in God.

__ I will have a baby, when God is ready.

__ I hate my life, when will I have a baby shower?

__ My body frustrates me because it will not do what I want it to do.

__ I want to hold my own baby, but I don't know if it will ever happen?

__ I am waiting for God to deliver my baby to me.

__ Baby clothes are so cute; I wish I had a child to buy for.

__ One day soon, I will shop in the maternity store

__ I wish God would hurry up and teach me whatever He wants me to learn.

Pray for God to make His Design for your life your Desire

Write a paragraph to God admitting whether your focus has been on your desires or on His design. Ask God for forgiveness if your desires have outweighed His design. Ask Him to reveal His design for you and your family. Seek God for help to realign yourself with His desire and ask for His will over your life and peace with His decision.

_____

_____

_____

_____

_____

_____

_____

_____

_____

_____

_____

_____

_____

_____

_____

_____ .

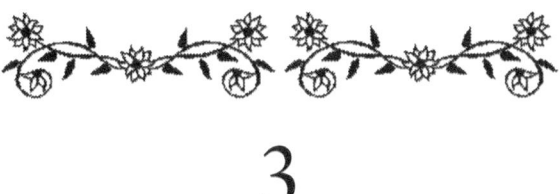

3

Determine to be Dedicated

---

1 Corinthians 15:58 Be steadfast, immovable, always abounding in the work of the Lord, knowing that your toil is not in vain in the Lord.

After traveling on the long stretch of road, *Desire vs. God's Design*, and purchasing our fruit and pecans, there is a rest stop ahead. The sign says, "Determined to be Dedicated." This is a perfect place to stop and rest from my long walk. As I sit on the benches, the beauty of the land quiets my spirit. The flowers are gracefully blowing in the air. This stop is different, there are others at this stop resting, but determined to complete their goals. Some are energized about their travel ahead; others look a little tired from the journey, but they are all determined to stay on the journey. You see, many on this journey are battling fear of the unknown, fear of what's ahead on the next road, and some fear of what they will do once they arrive on that road. But they all are functioning with one mind; they are determined to be dedicated to the end. Each knows they must first believe in their heart, make their determination a reality in their mind, and then establish it with their actions.

Write these scriptures and replace the blank with your name. For the next twelve weeks, take these scriptures memorize and meditate on them day and night.

1. *Jeremiah 29:11—For I know the plans I have for _____, declares the Lord, plans for welfare and not for calamity to give _____ a future and a hope.*

2. *Psalms 128:3—_____shall be like a fruitful vine within my house, _____'s children like olive plants around my table.*

3. *Psalms 46:1—God is _____'s refuge and strength, a very present help in the time of trouble.*

4. *Philippians 4: 13—I (_____) can do all things through Him who strengthens me.*

5. *Psalms 113:9—He makes _____abide in the house as a joyful mother of children. Praise the Lord.*

6. *Mark 11:23—Truly I say to _____, whoever says to this mountain, "Be taken up and cast into the sea and does not doubt in her heart, but believes that what she says is going to happen, it will be granted to _____.*

7. *Mark 11:24—Therefore I say to you, all things for which _____ prays and asks, believe that _____ has received them and they will be granted to _____.*

8. *Psalms 127:3—Behold children are a gift of the Lord, the fruit of _____'s womb is a reward.*

9. *1 John 4:4—You are from God, little children and have overcome them, because greater is He who is in _____ than he who is in the world.*

10. *Philippians 4:6—Be anxious for nothing, but in everything by prayer and supplication with thanksgiving let _____'s requests be made known to the Lord.*

11. *1 Corinthians 6:19—_____'s body is the temple of the Holy Spirit who is in _____, whom _____ has from God, and that _____ is not her own?*

12. *Isaiah 41:10—Do not fear for I am with _____; do not anxiously look about you, for I am _____'s God. I will strengthen _____, surely I will help _____, surely I will uphold _____ with My righteous right hand.*

Fortify your mind with the Word of God, so that you will be determined to be dedicated throughout this journey.

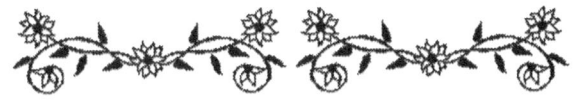

In addition to working on your mind, you have to also work on your body. I wanted to lose weight, so I drank 48-64 ounces of water a day, ate plenty of fruit and vegetables, and exercised at least 3 times a week. This is a good routine if you need to lose weight or if you don't. Start first by following the nutrition guidelines which list the proper servings of healthy foods. One way to start your healthy routine is to record everything you eat for a week, this will help to determine your eating patterns. Make several copies of the nutrition journal below, and record your eating and exercise patterns for the span of seven days. As always, check with your physician before you begin.

Nutrition Journal

Day _____

Breakfast

Snack

Lunch

Snack

Dinner

Water (8oz glasses) 1 2 3 4 5 6 7 8 9 10 11 12

Exercise: Yes   No

Types of exercise: Walking   Treadmill   Weights   Bike   Swimming

4

Doubting→Disappointment→ Desertion

Hebrews 13:5-6, I will never desert you nor will I ever forsake you. So I will con-fidently say, The Lord is my helper I will not be afraid.

Well, I guess I have rested long enough. I've had the opportunity to take in the scenic beauty of God's great land and partake of my apples. I must continue forward on my journey. My directions tell me to take a right at the next road sign, but I think I should probably take a left. For some reason, the road to the right, doesn't look like the best way to go, so I'll turn left here. If this takes me in the wrong direction, I can always make a U-turn. As I travel down this road, it looks unfamiliar as well. This road is a lot narrower and darker than the "Road to Fruitfulness." As a matter of fact, the trees are so close together, this looks more like a forest instead of a regular roadway. I doubted my directions, and now I am disappointed with the place I find myself. Once more, I feel deserted, there is no one around, I hear voices but I don't see anyone.

In your own words, define the word doubt

_____

_____.

List (3) three reasons people doubt.

1. _____
   _____
   _____.

2. _____
   _____
   _____.

3. _____
   _____
   _____.

Write the scripture James 1: 6-8

_____
_____
_____
_____
_____
_____
_____
_____
_____
_____.

Do you think God is pleased when we doubt? Why or why not?

_____
_____
_____
_____.

Refer back to "The Making of a Joyful Mother" and write down two reasons doubting is dangerous.

1. _____
   _____.
   _____
2. _____
   _____
   _____.

Who wants and even likes us to doubt more than anyone else?
a) God   c) Satan   e) Family
b) Self   d) Friends

| Doubting is an invitation for Satan to enter into our minds |

Match the verses with the correct scripture reference

1. Why do doubts arise in your hearts?   _____ Psalms 37:4
2..... He will give you the desires of your heart. _____ James 1:6
3.... does not doubt in his heart but believes ... _____ Luke 24:38
4. But he must ask in faith without any doubting   _____ Mark 12:23
5. God calls into being that which does not exist   _____ Romans 4:17

Write down (5) five areas in your life where you desire something, but sometimes doubt if you will receive it. These are areas where you need God to speak to your situation. I will give you the first one.

1. Healthy baby boy or girl
2. _____
3. _____
4. _____
5. _____

If God can speak and cause the heaven and earth to come into existence, then what can He speak into your life. Just because you cannot physically see the victory does not mean you won't have the victory. Do you realize that many of us have more faith in the natural world than we do in the spiritual world? This is a complete contradiction. The spiritual world caused the natural world to come into being. You have to start seeing yourself blessed and favored before you receive the blessing and the favor.

When _____ festers, it gives birth to _____, _____ gives birth to _____. Refer to "The Making of a Joyful Mother" book, Chapter 4.

Fearful contemplation means to be indecisive about venturing forward due to an event or a situation that has caused us pain or hurt in the past.

List (3) three things you are fearful of:

1. _____
2. _____
3. _____

Faithful contemplation means a positive reflection on Gods' goodness in your life.

List (3) three things you have faith in:

1. _____
2. _____
3. _____

Read and write 1 John 4:18

_____

_____

_____.

Review all six responses and ask yourself why there is fear in some areas and faith in God in others. Use this exercise to increase faith in the areas where fear is present.

List how you can turn fear into faith for the areas listed under fear.

1. _____
2. _____
3. _____

Write down your feelings of doubt, disappointment and desertion and find scripture references to replace these feelings with God's grace and love.

Feelings of Doubt	Scripture Reference

Feelings of Disappointment	Scripture Reference

Feelings of Desertion	Scripture Reference

This exercise is to make you mindful of your feelings and thoughts that often-times accompany infertility. I want you to overcome these feelings and thoughts with scripture references. The Word of God comforts and pours encouraging feelings and thoughts into your spirit instead of negative ones. Allow God and His Holy Spirit to minister to you; don't hide these feelings because God already knows about them. Instead, approach His throne openly and honestly, allowing Him to soothe your hurts and pains in the way that only He can do.

5

Decisions

Psalms 119:133—Establish my footsteps in Your word,
and do not let any iniquity have dominion over me.

I am lost, I mean really lost. Should I turn around and get out of this forest, or do I keep going, hoping to run into a street that will connect me back to the "Road to Fruitfulness." I don't know what to do. Maybe I should have taken the right turn like the map said. With the amount of time I have wasted, I could have been in the Daddy & Daughter section of town by now. Maybe I should go back the way I came, or can I even figure the way back? Everything looks the same. I need to face it; I made the wrong the decision. How do I get back on the right road?

Decisions are a very important part of all of our lives. The decisions we make today subsequently effect our tomorrow. That is why we have to be very careful about the decisions we make. They have either a positive or negative outcome. However, there are times when we make a decision (for example to have a baby) and for various reasons, that decision does not manifest itself when and how we would like for it too. So, we must go back and review our decisions. We first have to begin with God, recognizing that He makes the ultimate decisions. With the understanding that <u>our decisions</u> are just that <u>our decisions</u>. Once we have this understanding, then we can go forward. *John 5:30 states, "I can do noth-ing on my own initiative* … This phrase is talking about Jesus submitting to God; that even Jesus recognizes that God is sovereign.

> Should I keep trying to get pregnant?
> Should I listen to my friends?
> Should I give up and stop trying?
> Should I adopt?
> Should I seek God?
> Should I take fertility drugs?
> Should I consider IVF?
> Should I continue to wait?
> Should I seek another doctor's opinion?

Because there are so many factors and emotions tied to our fertility, we have tons of questions that need to be answered and lots of decisions to make. However, there is one decision that we should not waiver on and that decision involves a submissive and willing spirit to be open to God's plan for us.

How do you feel about God when God's plan for your life is different than your plan for your life? Circle all that apply

a) upset   b) angry   c) disappointed   d) happy

How do you respond to God when God's plan for your life is different than your plan for your life? Circle all that apply

a) accept God's will   b) reject God's will   c) indifferent

What is your thought toward God's plan?

_____

_____.

Do you think your plan is better than God's plan? Why?

_____

_____

_____

_____

_____.

How do you think God feels when He has made a decision for your life and you are displeased with His decision?

_____

_____

_____

_____.

List the decisions you have made regarding your infertility

1. _____

2. _____

3. _____

Did you make these decisions independent of God or dependent on God?

_____

Every situation that occurs in your life is predestined and ordained by God. The great thing about God is that He already knows the decisions you will make. But can you be submissive to God's decisions even when they are not your own?

What has God spoken to you, regarding your infertility?

_____

_____

_____.

If God has not spoken to you regarding your infertility, have you talked with Him?

_____

_____

_____.

We are not placed on this earth to fulfill our own agendas; we are placed on this earth to glorify God only. The Bible states in *1 Corinthians 6:20, For you have been bought with a price: therefore glorify God in your body.*

Define joyful:

_____

_____.

Define fruitful and multiply:

_____

_____

_____.

List (5) five ways you can be fruitful and multiply with children not born from your womb.

1. _____

2. _____

3. _____

4. _____

5. _____

Because God is all knowing and powerful, He can answer our prayers immediately, but have you ever thought about why God is not answering our prayers immediately?
Could it be that He wants us to be fruitful and multiply without giving birth?
Can you be open to God's will even if it's not what you planned?

Adopting is giving birth from the heart

Are you open to adoption? _____
If not, why?

_____
_____
_____.

Read the story of Moses & Pharaoh's daughter in Exodus, Chapter 2
What do you think would have happened to Moses if Pharaoh's daughter had not adopted him?

_____
_____
_____.

How would Moses' life have been different living with his natural mother?

_____
_____
_____.

What benefits did God give Moses' natural mother?

_____

What benefits did Moses receive as the son of Pharaoh's daughter?

_____

_____.

What benefits did Pharaoh's daughter receive from the adoption of Moses?

_____

_____.

What was Moses' God—given purpose for his life?

_____

_____

_____.

What did this adoption of Moses eventually do for the children of Israel?

_____

_____.

Whose agenda was more important to God?
a) Moses'   b) Pharaoh's daughter
c) Moses' natural mother   d) Pharaoh's   e) God's

In this story, all of the needs of Moses, Pharaoh's daughter, and Moses' natural mother were met. Moses was brought up with love, education, skill, and training that provided the ability to free his people. Pharaoh's daughter was allowed to pour her love and care into Moses which in turn blessed them both, because she did not have a child. Moses' natural mother was blessed because her son's life was spared. By living in Pharaoh's house, he was safe from harm and would be raised with all of the necessities and luxuries that his natural mother could not provide. Additionally, Moses' natural mother was even allowed to nurse her son as an infant, even though no one in Pharaoh's house knew she was Moses' natural mother. She continued to be a part of his life and could watch him grow into a man. Finally, God's plan to free the children of Israel from bondage was accomplished by using Moses. You see, it all works perfectly when we submit our lives to God and He determines how and why His ultimate plan must be accomplished. But in the end, you don't lose, you win because He makes sure that in the process and after that your needs are being met the way He intended. Submitting your will to the Father is always a "win win" not a "lose lose."

How would you feel if part of God's agenda is for you to adopt?

_____

_____.

Would you embrace His agenda or reject it?

_____

_____.

List (3) three important things you can provide an adopted child.
1. _____
2. _____
3. _____

> *Hopefully, you see why God's agenda is so much more important than our agenda. God accomplished freeing a whole nation by using Moses. The adoption of Moses into Pharaoh's house was an integral part of God's plan for Israel. What integral part do you play in God's plan for His kingdom?*

 Read these scriptures and answer the following questions.
Just as He chose us in Him before the foundation of the world, that we would be holy and blameless before Him.
In love He predestined us to adoption as sons through Jesus Christ to Himself, according to the kind intention of His will,…. Ephesians 1:4-5

In the scripture above, who is it referring to when it says "He?"

_____

Who is the scripture referring to with regards to "we?"

_____

In your own words, define the word chose:

_____

What was the purpose of God choosing us?

_____

In your own words, define predestined?

_____

_____.

What is the act of God that places the believer in His family?

_____

_____.

It involves a choice on whose part? _____

According to Psalms 119:133, how are our footsteps established?

_____

Many of the avenues and roads we take, we should not be on. If we would only consult God first, we would be spared much of the heartache that our own decisions can cause. However, we cannot begin to do so without reading and applying God's word to our lives. Some of us have made up our own minds about the best strategy for obtaining a baby and are now dealing with the consequences of that decision—depression, disappointment, hopelessness. But He wants us to seek Him, and He can remove all of the mental and physical ailments that are holding us back from being a "Joyful Mother."

6

The Deceiver

Revelations 12:9—".... Satan who deceives the world"

I have been walking for what appears to be hours to me, and I am still lost. Everything I see: trees, bushes and grass, it all looks the same. How did I get on this road? I'm not sure that I even know. Every time I make a turn, I seem to find myself farther and farther away from my intended destiny. I did talk to someone who I thought could help me find my way out of this maze, but that too was disturbing. He told me that I was on the right track, and I explained how I had doubted and was greatly disappointed by my experience. So much so, that I had come to the point of feeling complete desertion. The whole time I explained my feelings to this stranger, he kept telling me not to worry that I was on the right track. In fact, he said there was nothing wrong with doubting; that it is actually good for the soul. Listening to him, I knew in my spirit that something was wrong, but I just could not pinpoint what exactly it was. He told me no matter what the signs say ahead to stay on this road. By the time we finished our conversation, I was not only confused but frustrated and wondered why I had shared my concerns with a complete stranger.

Who is the deceiver? Many may think anyone can be a deceiver, and this is a correct assumption. However, there is only one deceiver that presides over all deceivers and all deception. His name is Satan, formerly known as "Lucifer" or some just call him the devil. Before Lucifer turned to the dark side, he was a beautiful angel created by God, residing in heaven and endowed with many

33

powers. But somehow, Satan got a little, shall we say, "full of himself" and saw himself as better than God, his creator. As a result, Lucifer convinced a third of the angels in heaven to join with him, just before God cast them into the abyss (Isaiah 14:19).

Let's look at how Satan is characterized in the Bible, so you will have a good understanding of this creature. Match the following by looking up the scripture and attaching the scripture to the name.

____ Murderer	a. Isaiah 14:12
____ Ruler of this world	b. Revelations 12:10
____ Devil	c. 2 John 1:7
____ Serpent	d. John 8:44
____ Adversary	e. Matthew 9:34
____ Prince of the air	f. John 12:31
____ Accuser	g. Ephesians 2:2
____ Deceiver	h. 1 Peter 5:8
____ Father of lies	i. John 8:44
____ Ruler of the demons	j. Matthew 4:1
____ Star of the morning	k. Genesis 3:1

How do you think Satan convinced a third of the angels to leave heaven?
(Isaiah, Chapter 14)

_____

_____

_____

_____

_____.

Has Satan told you any lies that would cause you to leave your God?

Circle Yes or No.

If yes, what has he said?

_____

_____

_____

_____

_____.

After studying the above and knowing what you know—Do you still believe Satan's lies? If so, why?

_____

_____

_____.

Satan told me (4) four lies during my struggle with infertility as outlined in "The Making of a Joyful Mother" book. Name each lie, he has told you.

1. _____

_____

_____

_____.

2. _____

_____

_____

_____.

3. _____

_____

_____

_____.

Satan gets into your mind and causes you to doubt yourself and God. His mission is to trick you into believing his lies about your destiny. He wants you to believe that your household will not be filled with beautiful children. He wants to silence your dream of tiny little feet running down the hallway. He wants you to believe that the sound of children's laughter will never be heard throughout your home. However, we must counter each and every lie thrown our way with the truth of God. We have to remember that God made us and God is based upon truth.

Write 2 Corinthians 10:5

_____

_____

_____

_____.

Listed below are feelings I felt during my struggle. Use this table to write scripture that refutes these feelings.

Worthless	James 1:4-
Alone	Hebrews 13: 5-6–
Envious	Job 11:18-

Name one lie that Satan has told you that relates to your past. Refer to "The Making of a Joyful Mother" Chapter 6

_____

_____

_____

_____.

Satan uses the emotions of embittered, guilt and embarrassed to cause us to questions ourselves and God. Write the below scriptures and memorize, so when the enemy brings your past before you. You can refute it with the Word of God.

Write Ephesians 4:22-23

_____

_____

_____

_____.

Write Psalms 32:5

_____

_____

_____

_____.

Write 1 John 1:9

_____

_____

_____

_____.

Write Philippians 3:13

_____

_____

_____

_____.

Write Romans 8:1

_____

_____

_____

_____.

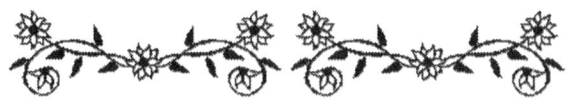

Part II

The Daddy & Daughter Relationship

Finally, up ahead to the right is the Daddy & Daughter Relationship Road. Oh thank God! I cannot wait to get on this street. I know that God is going to use this road to give me warmth, security and truth. I am not even on the street yet, but I can feel God's warm embrace. How did I ever get lost and travel down roads that provided me no edification or encouragement. Well, I cannot dwell in the past. I must look forward to God's amazing love and His future for me. As I am approaching, the Road to Fruitfulness merges into the "Daddy & Daughter Relationship". I will never deviate off of this road again.

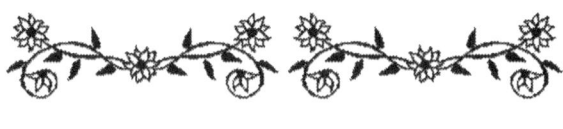

7

God Loves His Daughters

1 John 5: 18—"We have come to know and have believed the love which God has for us. God is love, and the one who abides in love abides in God, and God abides in him.

Search the Bible and find (3) three verses and their references that discuss God's love for us. If you don't know where to look, look in a concordance or index at the back of your Bible.

Scripture Reference   Scripture

1. _____

2. _____

3. _____

Look up John 3:16-17 and write it below.

_____

_____

_____

_____

_____

_____

_____.

What was God's ultimate sacrifice for us?

_____

_____.

Why do you think He allowed His Son to die?

_____

_____.

Who does God love?

_____

Circle all that apply. The world involves who?

Me   You   Our friends Our enemies   The Rich   Females
Doctors   Handicapped   Teachers   African-Americans   Preachers
Men   Atheists   Caucasians   Girls   Muslims   Child Molesters
Women   Homosexuals   The Poor   Hispanic-Americans   Children
Thieves   Lawyers   Asian-Americans   Murderers   Heterosexuals
All races & nationalities, all occupations/vocations—everyone on the face of
the earth

What does God require you to do to have eternal life?

_____

_____.

What do you gain if you accept Jesus Christ?

_____

_____

_____.

What happens if you reject God's gift, Jesus Christ?

_____

_____

_____.

Do you love God more than your desire to have a baby? Why or why not?

_____

_____

_____

_____.

Can you still love God, if He chooses not to answer your prayer the way you want Him to? If not, why?

_____

_____

_____

_____.

Seedtime/Harvest Time Principle:

This principle is explained on page 69 of "The Making of a Joyful Mother" and bears reviewing before completing this exercise.

List the names of (3) three children you have poured love into this year.

1. _____

2. _____

3. _____

List (3) three acts of love you have poured into these children this year.

1. _____
2. _____
3. _____

If all of these spaces are blank, then the seedtime/harvest time principle is not active in your life. Start with a small token; it does not have to involve money. Volunteer to baby sit for a mother, visit an orphanage, or bake some cookies and take them to a women's shelter. There are so many ways that you can share and show love to children, but it takes time and effort to do so. Remember the scripture *Matthew 18:5, whatever you do to the least of these you do it unto me.* God sees and hears all.

Record what acts of love you plan to pour into a child this month.

_____
_____
_____
_____
_____
_____.

Exercise: For the next nine months, find a child and/or children whom you can pour acts of kindness and love into each month and record your seed sowing below.

Name of Child	Month	Acts of Love/Kindness
1._____	_____	_____
2._____	_____	_____
3._____	_____	_____
4._____	_____	_____

5._____   _____   _____
6._____   _____   _____
7._____   _____   _____
8._____   _____   _____
9._____   _____   _____

After sowing your first seed, spend some time journaling what you did with the child, how you felt and what impact you made on this child. Spending a little time with a child serves a threefold purpose: 1) It demonstrates to God that you are willing to serve another by giving time, effort and energy, 2) It gives the child an opportunity to feel loved and cared for by someone other than their parent and 3) It gives you practice while you await your bundle of joy to be delivered to you.

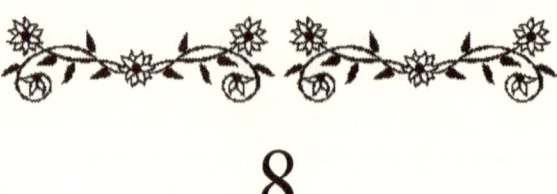

8

God Protects His Daughters

1 Peter 1:5-.... who are protected by the power of God through faith

God is such a protector of His children. He protects us from so many different scenarios that could happen in our lives. He even protects us from ourselves. You may be thinking, "But how?" Oftentimes on the journey of infertility, many of us develop negative thoughts about ourselves, our bodies, our husbands and even our God. Instead of allowing us to wallow in our thoughts, God seeks to protect us by reminding us of His love through a friend, a kind word, or by speaking a quiet word of hope into our situation. I am sure you have heard that old saying, "You are your worst enemy." Well, that's because God knows that He has to protect us not only from outside influences, but also inside influences, mainly ourselves.

Read and write Proverbs 23:7

_____

_____.

What does this verse mean?

_____

_____.

List (3) three positive thoughts you've had regarding your infertility

1. _____
   _____
   _____.

2. _____
   _____
   _____.

3. _____
   _____
   _____.

How many times a week do you think positive thoughts about your infertility?
a) once   b) two-three times   c) every day   d) almost never

List (3) three negative thoughts you've had regarding your infertility.

1. _____
   _____
   _____.

2. _____
   _____
   _____.

3. _____
   _____
   _____.

How many times a week do you think negative thoughts about your infertility?
a) once   b) two-three times   c) every day   d) almost never

If you are thinking negative thoughts every day or most of the week, then you must change your mindset. Remember our scripture "as a man thinks, so is he." As we analyze our thoughts, we recognize when we think negative thoughts, these thoughts fester and eventually come out of our mouth as words. Words affirm our thoughts.

Read and write Proverbs 18:21

_____
_____
_____ .

Have you spoken life over your womb? Yes or No
If yes, write what you have spoken

_____
_____
_____
_____ .

If no, write what you have spoken

_____
_____
_____
_____ .

If no, are you ready for the consequences of your spoken words?

_____
_____
_____ .

Circle all the phrases that bring life to your womb.

God is blessing me   It will probably never happen Why me?

I have so many problems God's timing is perfect   I am a joyful mother

My body is blessed   My mind is focused on God I don't care anymore

I am sick of waiting   I have chosen names for my babies

Your Choice

> Words of defeat spoken over your body and its'
> ability to reproduce will produce death

Vs.

> Words of victory spoken over your body and its
> ability to reproduce will produce life

Maybe some of you have spoken death over your womb unintentionally, not realizing the power that our words hold. If this is the case, don't panic, because we serve a God who is gracious and abounds in mercy. Let's go back to God's Word and find out how we can fix this dilemma. The Bible states in *2 Corinthians 10:5, "we are to take every thought captive to the obedience to Christ."* This can be a difficult task, but every time we think or say a negative thought, we must retract it and replace it with a positive thought or saying. We must learn to walk this journey of infertility by using positive thoughts to fuel our faith while expecting God to show up in our situation.

Write a vow to the Lord explaining that you will speak life to your situation and not death. Tell God, how you plan to execute that vow?

I (_____) vow to:

_____

_____

_____

_____

_____

_____

_____

_____.

Seedtime/Harvest Time Principle:

You may not be able to protect all children, but you can pray for their protection. If you are asking which children should I pray for, pray for children that you know as well as those you don't know. Be specific in your prayer; pray for the protection of all the children that have been abducted, all children in schools, all children in abusive family situations, homeless children and those in foster care.

List the names of three (3) children or three (3) categories of children you are praying for—with regard to their protection.

1. _____
2. _____
3. _____

We know from reading God's Word that prayer is a powerful tool; in fact He states that we must *pray without ceasing*. Praying for a child's protection places a Godly safety net over his/her life and brings you one step closer to the Father.

9

God Provides for His Daughters

Philippians 4:19 states that "God will supply all your needs according to His riches in glory in Christ Jesus."

Many focus on this scripture for financial reasons, but the scripture states that He takes care of <u>all</u> of our needs. For this chapter, we are going to focus on our emotional needs and well-being and see how God nurtures us as His children.

Name (3) three ways God has nurtured and comforted you, when you have encountered difficulty other than infertility.

1. _____
2. _____
3. _____

Has God nurtured you during this time of infertility? Yes or No

Explain how?

_____
_____
_____
_____.

One way God nurtured me during my trial was through prayer. Talking to God was healing for me because it allowed me to get my concerns and problems out into the open with God. I could be real with Him about how I felt and I did not have to feel ashamed or be ridiculed for feeling the way I felt. It also allowed me to shift the burden of infertility from me carrying it to God carrying it.

Read and write Matthew 11:28-29

_____
_____
_____
_____
_____
_____.

What is God asking us to do, when He asks us to "Come to Me?"

_____
_____.

Define weary:

_____
_____.

> ## *"Weariness makes you tired and causes you to lack hope and eventually stop believing that God can really bless you with a baby."*

Define heavy-laden

_____
_____.

What does God tell us about His yoke?

_____

What does that mean to you?

_____

_____

_____.

What actions are you going to take to rid yourself of worries and anxieties and take on God's rest?

_____

_____

_____

_____

_____

_____.

Philippians 4:6 states, If you draw close to Him, He will draw closer to you.

List (2) two ways you can draw closer to Him.

   1. _____

      _____

      _____.

   2. _____

      _____

      _____.

What do you think will be the benefit of you drawing closer to Him?

_____

_____

_____.

How will drawing closer to God benefit you during your journey through infertility?

_____

_____

_____

_____

_____

_____

_____.

Write a prayer to God asking Him to teach you to exchange your burdens for His yoke and instruction on how to draw closer to Him during this time of infertility.

_____

_____

_____

_____

_____

_____

The second way that God nurtured me during my struggle with infertility was through the Word of God. This type of spiritual nurturing is a vital component in developing and maintaining a relationship with God. In addition to a relationship with God, the Bible answers every situational question in life. However, many of us truly don't believe this. For example, is infertility or barrenness really addressed in the Bible? Let's look and see.
I invite you to read these passages of scripture because they demonstrate that you are not alone and that this is not a new struggle.

Examples of infertility in the Bible:

Abraham (100 years old) & Sarah (90 years old)–Isaac {Gen 11:30}

Isaac (60 years old) & Rebekah–Jacob & Esau {Gen. 25:21}

Jacob & Rachel–Joseph {Gen 30}

Elkanah (Great grandson of Esau) & Hannah–Samuel {1 Sam 1:19}

Manoah's wife–Judges 13

Zacharias & Elizabeth–John {Luke 1: 5-8, Luke 1: 36-37}

The third area God used to nurture me was meditation. Meditation involves hearing from God. It involves sitting quietly with God's Word and listening to how it applies to our situation. Meditation takes time and effort because there are so many distractions that take our attention from our inner thoughts. Many of us are so busy oftentimes; we don't have time to sit quietly and listen to our thoughts or a thought that God places in our minds. You might be thinking, "How do I meditate? Where do I start?" Well, first find a quiet place and allow yourself to be calm. Let yourself relax by breathing deeply and closing your eyes. Now listen to the voice of God. Before you begin answering the below questions, take some time now and truly meditate and listen for a still small voice, that's voice of God.

What thought was spoken into your spirit?

_____

_____

_____

_____.

When we are still, quiet and open to God's voice, there is a multitude of revelation that God will pour into our spirit which guides and directs our lives, if we listen to it?

As I stated earlier, there are many distractions that can cause our minds to wonder onto other things: such as doing the dishes, answering the phone, and/or running a quick errand. Oftentimes, our flesh wants us to focus on everything else in life, but the spirit. *Galatians 5:17 states, for the flesh sets its desire against the Spirit and the Spirit against the flesh; for these are opposition to one another, so that you do not do the deeds that you please.*

Now let's take this a step further, read *Jeremiah 29:11 which states, For I know the plans I have for you; plans for welfare and not for calamity to give you a future and a hope.* Look intently at the words of this scripture and ponder their meaning. Now, close your eyes and think/meditate on this scripture.

Write down what you heard God speak to you regarding your future?

_____

_____

_____.

Meditation is a great way to hear from God. Use meditation to find out God's plan for your family. Whether we like it or not, God teaches us through trials. If you read the stories in the Bible of those facing infertility, God is teaching through the trial. For some of us, God uses infertility as a teaching tool, and as a result, we have to examine our situation and our relationship with God to determine what He is trying to teach us in the midst of our trial.

Do you know what God is trying to teach you about your infertility?

_____

What do you think God is trying to teach you with regard to infertility?

_____

_____

_____

_____.

Barrenness is defined as being without a child, sterile or that which cannot produce offspring. In your examination of barrenness, focus on two factors: 1) What am I without? Is the answer to this question faith in God, love for my fellow man, true contentment, etc? You have to determine for yourself what you are lacking.

2) What is it that I need to be without? Hatred toward a co-worker and/or jealousy of a friend. Meditate on this concept and really search your soul for answers to these questions.

Are there any areas of your life that are barren?

_____
_____
_____.

What do you need to be without? What are you going to do to rid yourself of these things?

_____
_____
_____.

Seed Time/Harvest Time Principle:

What can you do to bless a child or children? There are many children in poverty stricken areas of the community that are in need of basic necessities all throughout the year, not to mention toys and clothing at Christmas. Some children need extra money for school field trips/activities and others need a blessing just to survive. We watch many children on TV suffer overseas because of lack food, water and clothing. There are so many opportunities for us to bless children; we all should be partaking in at least one.

List (3) three ways you plan to bless a child or children this year.

1. _____
2. _____
3. _____

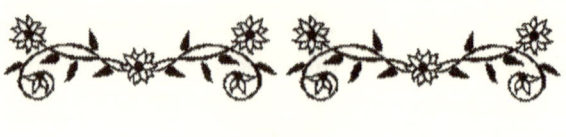

10

God Speaks to His Daughters

Deuteronomy 5:24—"... we have heard His voice from the midst of the fire; we have seen today that God speaks with man ..."

As women, we love to talk to our girlfriends, mothers and others about our problems; all in the hope that they will provide us with some answers and/or encouragement to help us get through our issue. Don't get me wrong, it's great for *iron to sharpen iron*, but calling our friends should not be the first step in resolving our issues.

How do you think God feels when you consult your friend's opinion before you consult His opinion? Check all that apply.

Happy	Disappointed	Insulted
Unhappy	Grateful	Pleased

God wants to be our Father and Friend. He wants to talk with us, but that cannot happen unless we talk and listen to Him daily.

Answer the following questions and write Father or Friend beside each statement that denotes a Father and each statement that denotes a Friend. Note, some may be both, so answer both.

_____ Provides for your needs/wants

_____ Loves us unconditionally
_____ Spends time talking about common interests
_____ Protects you from hurt, harm and danger
_____ Someone to call when you are in need
_____ Gives great gifts
_____ Has to discipline His children

Complete this scripture

1 Peter 5:7 states, Cast _____ of your _____ upon Him for He_____ for _____.

In **The Making of a Joyful Mother**, I explain the ways that God speaks to me; list the ways God has spoken to you:

1. _____
2. _____
3. _____

If you are not hearing from God, then it is time to examine your relationship with Him. First, you must begin by reading His Word and praying to Him daily. A relationship must be established before you are able to hear the voice of God.

John 10:27 states, "My sheep hear My voice, and I know them and they follow Me."

This is a powerful statement because it acknowledges that He speaks to His people, and they in turn hear His voice. So, there is no question, God does speak to His people. If we are not hearing from Him, it is our job to find out why. One way you can begin hearing from God is through His Word. Read God's Word and meditate on it, over and over, and listen for God's voice.

Oftentimes you will question if you heard His voice or yours, but keep reading and meditating and listen. You may be thinking, "How long do I meditate? I have not heard anything." Continue to meditate until you hear from Him.

After studying your Bible, began to research the names of God. Match the names with their meanings using the reference beside each statement.

_____ El Elyon	a. The Lord is Peace (Judges 6:24)
_____ Jehovah Jireh	b. The Lord is my shepherd (Psalm 23:1)
_____ Jehovah Raah	c. Lord (Master) (Joshua 5:14)
_____ Adonai	d. God Almighty (Genesis 17:1)
_____ Elohim	e. The Lord will provide (Genesis 22:14)
_____ Jehovah Shalom	f. Most High (Genesis 14:22)
_____ Abba	g. Father (Mark 14:36)
_____ El Shaddai	h. Strong One (Genesis 1:1)
_____ Emmanuel	i. God with us

It would be a good idea to familiarize yourself with the names of God, in fact choose one name each week and meditate on the name and its meaning for your life, watch God minister mightily to you. God is so pleased when we seek knowledge and a relationship with Him.

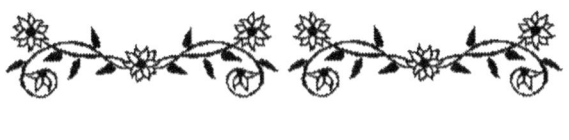

11

God Forgives His Daughters

Psalms 79:9—"Help us, O God our salvation for the glory of Your name; and deliver us and forgive our sins for Your name's sake."

Many of us have been praying for years for a beautiful, healthy baby. But for many, those prayers have not been answered. As a result, we have become overwhelmed with our circumstances and have somewhat resorted to anger with and against God. This is not a healthy exercise for you, and it does not help your relationship with God.

Are you mad at God because He has not answered your prayers? _____.

If yes, explain your feelings?

_____
_____
_____
_____.

Have you dishonored God because He has not answered your prayers for a baby? _____

If so, how?

_____

_____

_____.

Write 1 John 1:9

_____

_____

_____.

What would our lives be like if God was mad at us or held a grudge against us?

_____

_____

_____

_____.

What if He decided He was upset and did not want to talk to us or spend any time with us, how would you feel?

_____

_____

_____

_____.

He forgives us even when we are mad at Him and blame Him for our circumstances. If you are upset with or even mad at God, please confess that right now and ask for His forgiveness because He is faithful to forgive. Let Him pour His precious love on you and shower you with His grace. God loves you and has a perfect plan for your life.

Unforgiveness is like a poison in your veins that affects every part of your life.

Seed Time/Harvest Time Principle:

Many of us choose to hold onto anger or unforgiveness towards another. Because unforgiveness is like poison, we need to find that person, address the issue and forgive them, as well as seek their forgiveness. Sow a seed of forgiveness and reap God's abundant forgiveness.

Is there someone that you need to forgive?

_____

_____.

Have you contacted them and forgiven them? If not, why?

_____

_____

_____.

Set a date and time you plan to call or visit the person you are harboring unforgiveness towards and watch God bless your obedience and faithfulness.

Name _____

Date _____

Time _____

Result of the meeting:

_____

_____

_____

_____

_____

_____

_____

_____

_____.

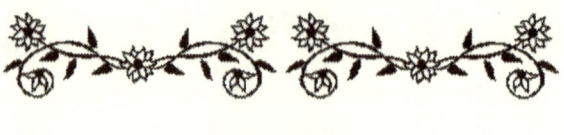

12

God Disciplines and Rewards His Daughters

Revelation 3:19 "Those whom I love, I reprove and discipline ..."
Psalms 58:11—"Surely there is a reward for the righteous."

Remember when you were a child and your mother or your father asked you not to do something, but you did it anyway? What happened? I'm sure he/she talked to you sternly, privileges were taken away from you, and/or you were spanked. God's response to us is similar to our parents' because He sets the model for parenting. If we truly desire to be parents, we must first master the role of a child.

What is the role of a child?

_____

_____

_____.

Does a child have the right to dictate to the parent what the parent should or should not give the child? If so, when?

_____

_____

_____.

Do you have the right to dictate to God when and how He should give you a baby?

Yes or No

Should parents automatically give their children what they want when they want it?
If so, what should be given and when should it be given?

_____

_____

_____

_____.

It's amazing how we understand the role of a child in relation to a parent, but we don't understand the role of a child in relation to the Heavenly Father. In society, our parents decided what we did and when we did it, but in life as adults, we think because we have reached the age of 18, we now decide what we do and when we do it.

> *And God wants us to understand that yes we have gotten a little older, but our role as His child has never changed. He is still God and we are still His children, and His agenda still overrides our agenda.*

What happens when we forget our role as children and God's role as parent?

We experience discipline   We experience reward

Write Revelation 3:19

_____

_____

_____

_____.

Write down one time you were disciplined by God and explain the discipline?

_____

_____

_____

_____.

How did you feel? Check all that apply

Upset   Sorry   Delighted   Confused   Happy   Mad

What did you learn from that experience?

_____

_____

_____

_____

What happens when we remember our role as children and honor God's role as parent?

We experience discipline   We experience reward

Write Psalms 58:11

_____

_____

_____

_____.

Write down one time you were rewarded by God and explain the reward.

_____

_____

_____

_____

_____

_____.

What did you learn from this experience?

_____

_____

_____

_____.

Seed Time/Harvest Time Principle:

Sow a seed into a child's life that has succeeded in accomplishing a task. Find a child who needs some encouragement and reward him/her. Everyone wants to feel like they are doing a good job. It doesn't have to be anything expensive, just give him/her a small token to let he/she know you are proud of him/her. We never know how something like this can change a child's life.

Name one thing you plan to do for a child this year that has completed a major accomplishment.

_____

_____

_____.

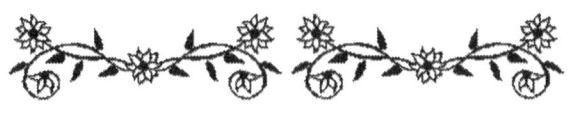

Part III

The Daughter's Arrival Into Destiny

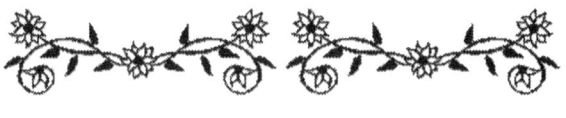

13

Driven to Dream

Daniel 2:3—"I had a dream and my spirit is anxious to understand the dream"

A dream is defined as experiencing thoughts, feelings, emotions, sounds, images and visions that occur during sleep. The great thing about dreaming is you never know when you will have a dream and what you will dream about. There is documented evidence that some dreams are prophetic in nature, providing exact and factual revelatory information to be fully revealed at a later time. Sometimes, a dream can cause us to overanalyze it to determine its meaning and whether the dream will come true or not. As we ponder the dream and its veracity, we see problems with the parts of the dream and wonder how they will be solved.

Define the word: problem.

_____
_____
_____
_____.

Define the word: opportunity.

_____
_____
_____.

During my trial of infertility, I began to dream and later see problems with my dreams. I had to make a conscious decision to see my problems with my dreams from a different perspective. Problems were no longer problems but actual opportunities for God to show up with His power and grace to perform the impossible in my life.

Let me give you an example of what I mean:

Dream: My husband and I are having dinner and enjoying one another's company. We love and respect one another deeply. I can't imagine my life without him. Everything is perfect.

Problem: My husband and I cannot see eye to eye on anything. We argue constantly, I am not sure that he even loves me anymore.

Opportunity: Father, I submit this marital turmoil to you. I am not sure as to why there is so much discord in our home, but I know you are faithful to change my heart and his heart, so that we compromise in love—always reflecting on You in our lives. So Father, I sit back and wait to see how You are going to bless this union that You put together.

Explain a dream you've had regarding having a baby.

1. _____
   _____
   _____
   _____
   _____.

List (3) three problems you see with the dream that you had.

1._____
2. _____
3. _____

Now take these (3) three problems and turn them into opportunities for God to bless you.

1. _____
   _____

2. _____

3. _____

Self Examination

Many of you have been walking on this journey of infertility for awhile, what have you learned about yourself in the midst of this trial?

What have you learned from others facing this same trial?

The first lesson I learned about myself and the trial of infertility was peace. Understanding and applying peace is the key to your whole being. Without peace in your life, you function in turmoil, disarray and uncertainty. Peace is a gift from God.

Write Ephesians 2:14

_____
_____
_____
_____.

In your own words, define: temporary peace.

_____
_____
_____
_____.

Now define: permanent peace.

_____
_____
_____.

You see, permanent peace cannot abide without God. In the book, **The Making of a Joyful Mother** I discuss temporary vs. permanent peace. Below list (4) four areas where you experience temporary peace.

1. _____
   _____
   _____.

2. _____
   _____
   _____.

3. _____
_____
_____.

4. _____
_____
_____.

Write John 14:27

_____
_____
_____
_____.

Write Philippians 4:7

_____
_____
_____.

The second lesson I learned during my struggle with infertility was in the area of contentment. For many of us, contentment is a hard place to find, because your feelings are in direct contradiction to being content. There are (4) four steps to arriving at contentment.

Step 1—Identify the problem

Write the problem down in the space provided

_____
_____
_____
_____
_____.

Step 2—Face the reality of the problem

(Acknowledge that you have done everything humanly possible in order for the problem to be solved).

_____
_____
_____
_____
_____.

Steps 1 & 2 demonstrate your thoughts, feelings and frustration with the problem

Step 3—Submitting the problem to God

_____
_____
_____
_____
_____.

Write Philippians 4:6

_____
_____
_____
_____
_____.

Fill in the blanks. Galatians 2:20

It is no longer _____ who live, but _____ who lives in _____.
The life which _____ now live in the _____ _____ live by
_____ in the _____ _____ _____, who loved _____ and
gave _____ for _____.

Pay very close attention to these verses because they take your focus off of you and your circumstances and place the focus on God and what He can do for you. I don't know what God's plan is for your life, but I know that He does everything for a reason. We have to stop focusing on what we want and start focusing on what He wants—it's not about us or our agenda, its' only about Him.

Step 4—Acknowledge God's sovereignty while you await your blessing

Write Colossians 1:16-17

_____

_____

_____

_____

_____

_____

_____.

What does this verse say about God and your infertility?

_____

_____

_____

_____.

Read Matthew 6:33 and fill in the blanks.

_____ _____ the kingdom of God and _____ _____and _____ these _____ will be _____ to _____. This verse acknowledges God's sovereignty.

Who has greater sovereignty in your life than God? Check all that apply
    your doctor   your best friend   your co-worker
    your husband   your mother   your pastor

You must seek God first above everyone and everything in your life. It is the only way to arrive at peace and contentment.

Can you say the statement below to God and mean it?
"If you never bless my womb, I will still praise you." It took me a long time before I could say this statement and mean it with all of my heart, but I did. I repeated it over and over to God, because I wanted Him to know I wanted a baby, but I wanted Him more.

The third lesson I learned was in the area of faith. Many are familiar with the verse in *Hebrews 11:1, Now faith is the substance of things hoped for, but the evidence of things that are not seen.* This means, even when you cannot see your blessing on the horizon, you know its coming, so you wait for it to show up at any moment. The problem with some of our faith is that if we don't see our baby soon, then we tend to stop having faith in this area. However, we must always have faith in what we don't see, unless God has said no to us. Remember earlier, we talked about God answering in one of three ways: 1) yes 2) no or 3) wait. Many are in the waiting period, so we must have faith until God answers.

Read Luke Chapter 1 and pay close attention to Luke 1:18-20
What did the angel of the Lord tell Zacharias concerning his family?

_____
_____
_____
_____.

What were the plans for Zacharias' son as spoken by the angel of the Lord?

_____
_____
_____
_____
_____
_____
_____
_____
_____.

After hearing the plans for his son, what did Zacharias ask the angel?

_____
_____.

What was the angel's response to Zacharias?

_____
_____
_____.

Why do you think the angel of the Lord made Zacharias mute?

_____
_____
_____
_____.

Write Hebrews 11:6

_____
_____
_____
_____
_____.

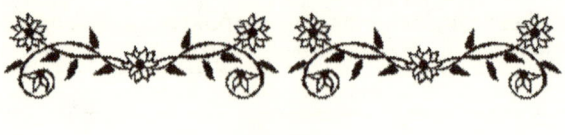

14

Defeating Difficulty

Jeremiah 32:27, "Behold, I am the Lord, the God of all flesh,
is anything too difficult for Me?

Pyramid of Faith

Level 4: Work your faith

Level 3: Grow your faith

Level 2: Stretch your faith

Level 1: Thicken your faith

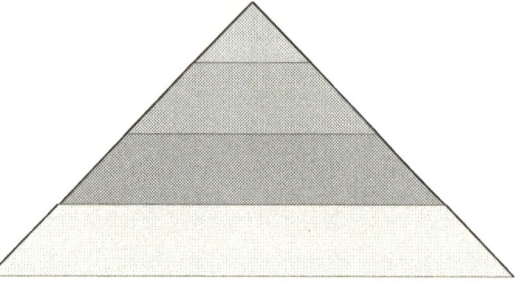

Faith is the key to defeating difficulty and it is the process by which we access God and His power. Begin to see your faith as a seed that is planted in the soil. As the seed is embedded in the soil, the seed thickens. The seed, your faith, is thickening by the Word of God, prayer and testimony. The environment around the seed changes, and as it is watered with the Holy Spirit, the seed (your faith) begins to stretch. As it stretches, it eventually bursts forward above the surface of the soil and sprouts forth visible for all to see. This "faith seed" has now transformed itself into a plant. As a plant, now your faith begins to grow. This is what your faith should be doing constantly. It should always be progressing forward. Because once it is full grown, then you can work your faith. For this chapter, we will focus heavily on Levels 1 & 2. If you can master the first two levels, Levels 3 & 4 become a breeze.

Level 1: Thicken your faith

Define the word: thicken—

_____
_____
_____.

Thickening involves layering. The goal is to layer your faith so thick that nothing can penetrate it—not illness, not disbelief, not a bad diagnosis, nothing. You may be thinking, "How do I thicken my faith?" As we have discussed in earlier chapters, you must have the Word of God and prayer. But in addition to these, a person's testimony can help thicken your faith.

Write Revelation 12:11

_____
_____
_____
_____
_____.

Explain how you can overcome by the word of someone else's testimony.

_____
_____
_____
_____
_____.

Write Acts 10:34

_____
_____

_____

_____.

Just in the last two months of completing this workbook, a 57 year old woman had her first baby, and before that, a 62 year old gave birth to a set of twins. That's layering your faith! Knowing that despite your current circumstances, God is still blessing others and can bless you as well. As you begin the exercise below, thicken your faith with testimony that is general and specific to your area—age, medical diagnosis, blocked tubes, hysterectomy. Whatever your issue is, there is someone who has faced the same issue and overcome it. You can find this information by researching the internet for articles, news stories, and any information you can find, even word of mouth testimonials. Copy and keep these testimonial nuggets in a place where you can find them.

Find one article or news story that discusses an unbelievable birth of a child and record it below.

_____

_____

_____

_____.

Level 2—Stretch your faith

Stretch your faith by opening up. So many women suffer in silence and they allow the trial of infertility to beat them down and eventually spiral them into a deep depression. One of the great gifts women have is talking to one another. I am not saying talk to everyone about your infertility, but there are avenues you can take part in to support you while you are on this road. There are infertility support groups on the internet, some hospitals have infertility support groups, and some support groups can be found online. Get connected to these groups, so you can share and discuss your feelings with women who are battling the same issue you are. Receive encouragement, and seek to give encouragement to one another. That's what sisterhood is all about. Oftentimes, these settings provide an environment filled with love and encouragement. If you feel that you are not ready to join a support group, contact an infertility/family counselor and meet one-on-one. The point is, don't go through this struggle alone.

List (3) three ways you are going to stretch your faith by opening up.

1. _____
2. _____
3. _____

As part of your stretching, begin to open up more with your husband. He is facing this issue too. I know you have probably tried talking to your husband and have become frustrated by his response or the fact that he does not see infertility the same way you do. But, I encourage you to go back to him and share your heart. Don't unload everything all at once, but gradually open up to him and discuss your concerns. A good practice for any married couple, but especially one facing infertility, is to pray together about this issue and then pray for each other in this area.

List (3) three areas of concern that you have not previously shared with your husband.

1. _____
   _____
   _____.

2. _____
   _____
   _____.

3. _____
   _____
   _____.

The last part of your stretching exercise involves your friends or relatives that are close to you. Ask friends and family to pray for your fertility, but also for your faith, emotional health and your physical well-being. Find friends and/or relatives that are faithful, prayful, mature, and sensitive. These are people that have your best interest at heart.

Let them know that this is a step toward stretching your faith in God.

List (2) names of people you will share your heart with.

1. _____
2. _____

By thickening and stretching your faith, you are well on the road to growing your faith. As long as you continue following the Word of God, prayer, and Levels 1 & 2, your faith will begin to grow exponentially. You will find yourself encouraging others while you are waiting for God to break forth the heavens and deliver your bundle of joy. Once your faith is fully grown, then you can begin to work your faith. Working your faith does not involve God being your puppet and you holding the string. Working your faith means that you and God have a relationship, and He sees you as His daughter, and you see Him as your Father. When there is a relationship between a daddy and a daughter, you know the daughter is the apple of her father's eye. He will sometimes do things for her that he would not normally do. This is the same principle with our Heavenly Father. He will grant grace when He should punish, or He will give mercy when He should take it away. God is such a great Father because He allows us to endure trials to teach us more about ourselves and more about Him. He then gives us a powerful testimony to share with others.

> *For many of us, we want to move past the process and go straight to the privilege, but it is in the process that the miracle of faith occurs.*

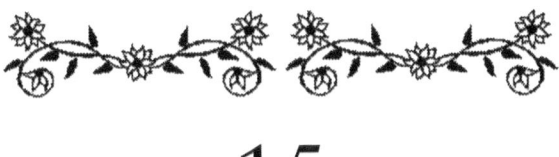

15

Destiny—Children of the Promise

Romans 9:8—It is not the children of the flesh who are children of God, but the children of the promise are regarded as descendants.

The miracle of my daughter was a visible sign to me that God could do anything. There is nothing too hard for Him. Through all of the ups and downs during my journey through infertility, I remain thankful for this trial. It's easy to want to rush through any trial to arrive on the other side, but without going through the process, we can miss out on the blessings that can only be taught in the storm. I have learned so much about God, about myself, and about the life-long valuable lessons He so patiently taught me.

You see, it was in this process, where God transformed me into a joyful mother.

Did God teach you anything new during your study of this workbook?

Yes or No

If yes, what did you learn?

_____

_____

_____

_____

_____.

Is your mind aligned with His will? Yes or No
If yes, explain.

_____

_____

_____.

> *I hope that you have enjoyed this study and I hope that it has brought you even closer to God. Be open to Him and His timing for your blessing. And realize, no matter what your situation is, He and He alone has the power to transform you into a joyful mother.*

978-0-595-43698-9
0-595-43698-6

www.ingramcontent.com/pod-product-compliance
Lightning Source LLC
Chambersburg PA
CBHW030406290526
45785CB00004B/1926